THE FINAL JOURNEY HOME

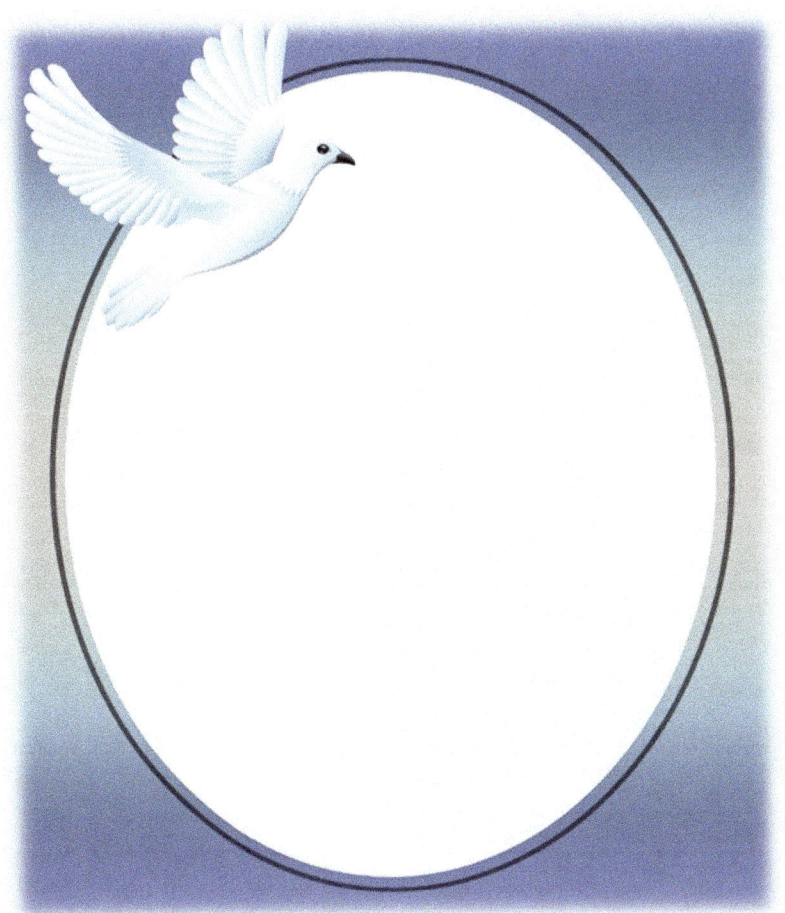

THE FINAL JOURNEY HOME

GLORIA MILLS BATTLE

First Printing: 2022

ISBN 978-1-387-85595-7

UNOME PUBLISHERS
PO BOX 1384, OWINGS MILLS, MARYLAND 21117

www.unomepublishers.com

Dedication

Alma Parks Mills

I dedicate this book to two special persons, Mrs. Alma Parks Mills (Mother) and my loving husband Garfield. These persons have made an impact in my life. My Mother was the joy of my life. She taught so much to carry me through for a life time. She laid the foundation for my life. I thank God for all of her love, her encouragement, and her words of wisdom. Even during her illness with Dementia, Mother still made us smile. Mother was a strong God fearing Woman; and she was my Hero. The wonderful memories of Mother will last for the rest of my life. Sadly Mom passed away peacefully in her home on April 7, 2017. I will forever hold Mother near and dear to my heart. I will always remember the great advice and words of wisdom she gave me. And we I don't recall anything else, I'll always remember Mother to me many times. Mother would often, to enjoy my life, and that what I'm going to try to do. My life won't ever be the same. Rest in Paradise Mother.

Garfield Battle

I would like thank my loving husband Garfield who has always been supportive during my Mother's battle with dementia. When Mother was first diagnosed Garfield stated that whatever I needed all I had to do was ask. I couldn't ask for a better husband than he. Garfield is a man of his word. I thank God for my wonderful husband who gave me words of encouragement and plenty of hugs when I need them. Garfield you are surely one of a kind. You gave so much of yourself to make sure that I was taken care of. I will be forever grateful for all that you are doing and have done for me. Garfield you are the love of my life and you bring me so much joy.

Contents

Introduction

One of the most important reasons I am writing this book is to help me and others during the healing process of losing a Mother or a family member to Dementia or Alzheimer's. It has been difficult losing my Mother to Dementia, and never in my wildest dreams, did I think that Mother would have to suffer through this disease in the prime of her life. It has hit me hard because she was diagnosed so early. The pain first begun when I received the news that she had Dementia. I felt like my heart had been broken into many pieces.

I was numb for months. I just wanted to be there by her side. The grief still remains, but I can handle it better today than I did five years ago. This book talks about the struggles of depression that I faced on most days. My message to you is that if you are going through grief, talk about your loved ones, pray for strength, and get professional help if needed. There is no time timeline on how long the grief will last. In this book I have included a chapter on the several stages of Dementia and grief as well.

I have always looked up to my Mother. We had a pretty good relationship in my younger days. Our relationship became better after I left home at 17 years old. She always gave me advice whether I liked it or not. We often spoke each week. In my single years, I traveled home often. Later on, when I got married, I didn't come home as often as I liked. Mother shared so much wisdom. When I did travel home to visit, we would spend time talking and sharing information. I could drive her over to visit her Mother; she always looked forward to visiting.

Most of the time, I always felt sad when I traveled back home from my visit. Many years ago, I made a promise to God to enjoy my parents in their younger days. I felt that when I traveled back to Maryland I would never know when it would be that last time I would see her. We shared so many memories that will last a lifetime. In writing this book, I hope that everyone will see that it's important to talk about death and grief. The grieving   process is different for everyone. You can allow it to cripple you, or you can work towards healing. My grief began the day when Mother was diagnosed with Dementia and by writing this book, it means that in time you and I will be able to move on and continue to heal from our grief.

When I wrote my first book, I felt a sense of relief and peace of mind. It was if the weight of the world had been lifted off of my shoulders. The joy came when I released some of the pain in dealing with the loss of Mother. I pray that by telling my story I will help someone that is going through some of the difficulties that I faced during my loss. Please know that you and I have an inner strength that we can tap into. One thing that you can do is to journal what you are going through from the beginning to the end. In my earlier book, I focused on the awesome memories of my love for my loved one.

Chapter 1: The Final Birthday Celebrations

Mother's Birthday Celebration:

- 89th- November 8, 2014
- 90th - November 9, 2015
- 91st -November 2016

The importance of my being able to attend Mother's birthday celebrations is that I realize that the months, days, and hours were numbered. I just wanted to be as close to her as I could to help her celebrate. I wanted her to be happy and enjoy her special celebrations. Due to her state of mind, she was there physically, but not mentally. It looks as if she did enjoy the celebrations while we were all together with her as a family.

Mother's 89th birthday was November 9th, but we celebrated it on November 8th in Greer. Most of the family traveled home to celebrate her birthday. We had a feast. We invited a few family members to attend the celebration. I dedicated the first book I wrote for Mother on that day.

Everything was in grand style. Mother held up well. We didn't keep her out too long. She didn't do well with a large crowd due to her condition with Dementia.

Mother's mood would change, and she would be somewhat difficult to handle; that was part of dementia. Even still, it was a great day. Mother celebrated two more birthdays before she passed away in 2017. I just thank God for the many birthdays that we celebrated with Mother. I didn't get to go home for Mom's 90th & 91st birthdays. Mother's condition had gotten worst so she didn't go out anymore. Mother spent most of her time in her lift chair and bed. By Mother's 90th birthday she was unable to walk. It was extremely difficult seeing Mother in her condition. It just broke my heart.

Chapter 2: Traveling Home

Mother's Day:

- <u>May</u> 1993 - May 2017

In the earlier years, I would rotate between Greer, S.C. and Rocky Mount, N.C. Many years I would travel to North Carolina to be with my husband for Mother's Day. I really missed visiting my Mother for Mother's Day. I thought that since I was married I needed to be with my husband and children. As time went by, my Mother-in-Law passed away in 1992. I started visiting my Mother every Mother's Day in 1993. I only missed one visit after that.

I was always happy to be there. I just enjoyed being around Mother. We shared some wonderful times. Mother would always give me something to take back home when I came to visit. I would tell her that she didn't have to do that, but that's what she wanted to do. Mother was a loving person, and she gave so much of herself. I do cherish those wonderful memories.   Mother would pass away before Mother's day in May of 2017.   I decided to return to pay tribute to her memory; it was a month after she passed away.

My first stop once I arrived home, after Mother's death in April 2018, was straight to the gravesite. I just couldn't hold back the tears.   It was difficult.   I'm still in disbelief, facing the reality of Mother being gone.   It was extremely difficult to go back home for Mother's Day, so I decided to travel back to celebrate the anniversary of her death each year.   Mother's Day won't ever be the same.   I will continue cherishing the wonderful memories that I have of Mother. I once heard that in time God will heal a broken heart.   I continue to dream about her. I think about her every day. I must trust God, he knows best.

Chapter 3: The Setbacks

Mother's setbacks are happening one after another and re are getting worse. The setbacks and her condition are getting worse one after another. I guess I was praying for a miracle. One day she would be doing okay, but the next day her condition would deteriorate even further. I would call several calls a day to check on Mother. Based on the different stages of dementia, I learned that with each stage Mother would get worst. I then made plans to travel home to South Carolina.

My siblings needed me to help take care of Mother. I couldn't help but to shed tears and feel very depressed. This visit would be different because Mother needed special care. I had to give her medication every two to three hours. I did my best to change her at night. It was extremely difficult to assist with her needs, but I did my best. I stood by Mother's bedside and prayed over her. Each time I came home, Mother was in a different stage of her Dementia.

Chapter 4: The End of Mother's Journey

The beginning of the end means facing the reality of
Mother's Death

- December 2016
- January– February 2017

At the end of December on New Year's Eve, I said a special prayer for my parents. Now it's a new year. I didn't know that this would be the year that would bring my Mother's journey to an end. It just broke my heart to think that my Mother's life was coming to end. It was February 2017 when I decided to travel back to South Carolina to assist with Mother's care. At the time I didn't realize that Mother was in the seventh and final stage of Dementia. I was still holding on, praying for a miracle.

Mother had developed an infection. It was so painful, just watching Mother waste away. Mother had lost so much weight. We had already been told by the nurse and social worker that if she didn't pass away from dementia, it would be something else. The next health issue with Mother would be pneumonia. Mother would come back each time, but I knew that she wouldn't get well. She took even more medicine. It was one health issue after another.

After about a week or so, I had to return back to Maryland. It was difficult for me to leave. I was always depressed when I returned. All I could do was to pray that God would allow Mother to be there when I returned back to visit her. I checked on her every other day. I realized that Mother wouldn't get well, and that the dementia would take her life. Before I left, I gave her a kiss, and told her that I loved her. I had always tried to hold back the tears, but I just couldn't.

Chapter 5: Finality

The Final Journey Home

March – April 2017

Before starting to write this part in the book, I have to take a deep breath and pray that God will hold back the tears. This is the most difficult chapter of my book that I have to write.

It's March and Mother's condition had gotten worst. The end was getting close. Mother's doctor decided to take her off of all of her medicine. The medicines were no longer helping her condition. This was the final confirmation that Mother would be leaving us and the only thing was that we didn't know when. I was a nervous wreck. I would pray each day that God would let Mother live long enough for me to see her at the end. My prayer has always been that when she finally dies, that she would go peaceful. God did grant my prayer.

As days went by, Mother would have another setback. My sister called me about 12:30am the night of March 27th to say that Mother has had a setback. This one was the worst. After this setback, Mother had to be put on oxygen to help her breathe. I didn't sleep at all that night. Everyone was upset. I spoke with the nurse after my I finished speaking to my sister. I cried and prayed all night. I couldn't wait until the next day.

As I recall this was the end of March. I didn't really know what I was going to do, stay here in Maryland or go back to see Mother for the final time. I prayed about the situation and spoke with my husband about my decision. I cried most of the day. I can recall it like it was yesterday. The day I received the news that Mother was worst was on a Tuesday, March 28th. It was final. I decided to travel back home to see Mother for the last time. I booked a flight for the last Wednesday in March. This would be one of the longest flights that I had ever taken home. I met a wonderful lady on the plane. She gave me words of encouragement when I told her that my Mother had dementia and had gotten worse. I tried my best to hold back the tears.

I arrived home safely. I went straight to see Mother. My Dad and my two sisters were there along with my cousin, who had been there helping take care of Mother. The first thing I did would be to go in to see Mother. I went into the room, then asked everyone to leave the room so that I could have some private time with Mother. I tried my best to be strong. It wasn't easy but I was calm. I gave Mother a kiss. She didn't open her eyes. The reality that Mother wasn't going to be with us much longer hit me hard.

I stayed with my cousin for a week before Mother died. I would travel back to our home each day. It was Wednesday night, April 5th and I stayed up all night watching over Mother. My cousin was there as well. Mother was so sick she couldn't stand for anyone to touch her. At the end she was in so much pain. On Thursday, April 6th, my niece came in from California. We were singing and praying over Mother. Mother reacted when my niece touched her. I was frightened for just short time. I couldn't bear the thought of Mother passing that evening. I ran out of the home because I thought Mother was passing away. The social worker told us that it would only be a matter of time that Mother would pass away.

Easter Sunday, the first Sunday in April, was the week before Mother passed away. I told Dad that he and my sister needed a break. I decided to stay home to take care of Mother. I was sure that she would pass away that Easter Sunday, but she didn't. Mother was getting weaker. I really just wanted to get in the bed with her to comfort her, but I didn't. I felt helpless. I wanted to tell her that I loved her. I bent down and kissed Mother. I told her in a soft whisper that I loved her. She replied to say that she loved me too.

Mother could still hear me. I felt so much joy. I just wanted to run around the house and shout out loud that she heard me. It had been said that the hearing is the last thing to go and that's true. That really made my day. It wasn't long before she wouldn't be able to eat or drink anything. It was difficult for Mother to swallow now. Mother lived one week without food or water and that was nothing but God. Mother was still holding on for something or someone. We continued to sing and pray over her.

I hadn't seen Mother's eyes since I arrived home. I prayed that God would allow me to see Mother open her eyes one more time. One of my sister's and I went shopping for a dress for Mother's homecoming service. I forgot my shawl, so I went back into the house to get it. I went back into the room to see Mother one more time she had her eyes open and was looking up at me. I told her that I loved her. I was so excited to get into the car to tell my sister that Mother had opened her eyes.

I had to go back to my cousin's house to get some rest. I came back to the house on Friday April 7th in the afternoon. One of my sisters and my cousin went out to take a break. I spoke to Dad. Then the social worker came in to speak with me. She showed me some signs that on this day, Friday, April 7th, would more than likely be the last day of Mother's life. In the meantime, Dad and my sister came into the room to see Mother. My sister asked Dad to sing Mother's favorite song. It was a song that Dad sang when he was in the church choir and my Mother loved for him to sing it.

Dad sang *"sat down servant, sat down, and rest a little while"*. All of us in the room were crying. After Dad sang, he and my sister went in the other room. The social worker said that when Mother started passing away it would be somewhat like when I'm on my CPAP machine; her chest would go up, but when the final time comes, Mother's chest would not come back down. I stayed there by her bedside checking on her heart rate and her breathing. I put my cell phone by Mother's ear so she could hear the gospel music that I was playing for her.

The social worker had gone in to speak with my sister. I continued checking Mother's breathing. When Mother took her last breath, I wasn't really sure so I bent down to see if I could feel her breath, but I didn't feel anything and no pulse. Mother had passed away while I sat there by her bedside. I didn't panic. The social worker was on her way to speak with Dad. I called her to Mother's bedside. I told her that I thought Mother had just passed away. She checked her pulse and heart rate. The social worker replied that Mother had passed. She asked me what the time was. I told her that it was 3:07pm. The social work told me that she had to wait until the nurse arrived again to call Mother's death.

After which the social worker went in to tell Dad and my sister. I stood on the other side of the bed. This was one hardest pill to swallow. The tears were rolling down my face. I just wanted to scream out loudly but I held it in. It wouldn't be long before my sister and cousin came back to the house to find out that Mother had passed away. This would be one day that I won't ever forget. I began to call my family members back in Maryland and local family to let them know that Mother had passed away.

Now that Mother had passed away it was time for the healing process to begin. We would start getting ready for Mother's homegoing service. We all wanted to get the arrangements finished as soon as possible. The family agreed not to have the service on a Sunday. So it was finished.

No more pain and no more suffering. Mother is now resting in paradise. I'll never forget April 7th, 2017. Sometimes I wonder why God chose me to be by Mother's bedside when she passed away. Maybe it was that God wanted me to be there to be strong, just like my Mother. Mother has always been my Hero. I really tried to be strong but inside my heart was broken. I couldn't wait until my husband and children and family arrived from Maryland. The funeral arrangement had been finished. Now I needed to prepare myself for what was coming.

The church was completely full that day. Mother was well loved. She had been a long-time member of the church. I felt so numb when the service started; it was if I was blocking everything and everyone out. After the funeral service, everyone was traveling back to their homes. Dad was suffering with grief as well. I just wanted to go back home but he needed me. I stayed there with Dad for one month. This was a difficult time for me. I'm thinking, "how can I be strong for anyone." I just wanted to go back to Maryland and grieve. There would be days when Dad and I just prayed for strength.

Afterwards, I returned back to Maryland. I did well until I returned home. That's when the grief began. I just couldn't hold back the tears. I cried for weeks.   I was in so much more pain. All I wanted to do was to stay in bed all day alone. I finally decided that I needed some professional help.   I made an appointment to speak with a therapist. It did help and I found that talking about Mother's passing was part of the healing process.

I spoke and talked to everyone that would listen. It would be several months before thinking about doing a book, sharing the difficulty of dealing with the death of a loved one. It has been almost five years since her passing. I still just take one day at a time. I won't ever forget Mother as long as I live. I do need to move on with my life and work on the purpose that God has planned for me but that hasn't happened yet.

Chapter 6: Dealing with Grief

Let not your heart be troubled: ye believe in God, believe also in me. In my Father's house are many mansions: If it were not so, I would have told you. I go to prepare a place for you. **John14 1-2 NIV**

I decided to write another book about facing the reality of Mother's death. Hopefully, this will help me deal with the grief and sadness that death brings. I watched Mother year after year, while her health was declining from dementia. Mother passed away, as I sat there by her side on April 07, 2017, at 3:05 p m. The struggle was real. As I begin to write this book, the tears begin to roll down my face. I think, "am I really ready to write this book"? I do pray that God will help me bring some closure to my life. At the time I tried to write this book, but I wasn't really ready. The pain of losing her was holding me back. I just couldn't do it.

It was as if when I started to complete the book, I became depressed all over again. It took me a while to regroup. Every time I told my daughter that I was ready for her to publish my book, I got more and more depressed. I see Mother's pictures everywhere. I'm missing Mother so much, but I thank God for the 91 years that he allowed her to be with us.

There isn't a day that goes by that I don't think about Mother. I pray that in time God will continue to give me strength to get through her death and bring some closure. I'm really trying my best to recover from the grief and sadness that I feel. In time God will heal my broken heart. In the beginning after Mother passed away, I felt as if I was blocking out her death. I was so busy doing what came from the heart, helping other family members deal with her grief.

I have always thought of myself, being like Mother, a strong woman. Sometimes, I feel like I don't have anyone to talk to but God. I'm leaning on God to help me through this grieving process. I know that Mother is looking down from heaven and she is smiling down on me. I thirst to see her again in a dream or a vision. The love is so deep that I have for my Mother still. Sometimes I think it's not real, and she just on a trip and will return. Mother always told me to enjoy life. I'm going to try my best to continue to get through this grief and sadness I had a close relationship with my Mother.

There will always be a void in my life, but in time the grief will get better.

Tribute to Mother's memory

April 2018 -1st year

Tribute to Mother's Memories

April- 2018 – April 2022

Many days, hours and months have passed.   April 7th, 2022 marks the 5th anniversary of Mother's death.   It has taken me a while to complete this book in memory of my Mother (Alma Parks Mills).   During this time there has been some healing, but it is still difficult for me to deal with her death. I have had a lot of sleepless nights just thinking about why she left me so soon. I do pray often,. but something is hold me back.   I finally realize the in order for me to heal and move on, it must let it go. I have seen her several times in my dreams. Most of the time the dream would take me back to my hometown of Greer. We have carried on a conversation; I recall in one of my dreams.   I really don't understand why these dreams keep coming to me. I recently saw an angel in my dreams, I thought maybe it was Mother, but I couldn't remember the face in the dream. It is if, my depression has gotten worst, due to Covid-19.

For what its worst, I'm still mourning the death of my Mother. Just the other day I awaken, feeling like I had a heavy burden on my heart. On that day, I just couldn't shake the depression. I signed on Facebook and read a prayer from one of my nieces. I knew that this prayer has for me. I have begun to feel better.

Just recently I decided to finish my book in memory of my Mother. I do feel like I can move on by here. Hopefully my book will help someone heal, and learn to deals with death. No, it's not going to be easy, but we can do it. Pray often and think of the things that will bring you Joy and Peace so that we can move on. With God's Grace and Mercy, we can do all things through Christ who strengthen us. Philippians 4:13

The month of April marks one year of the Mother's death. She passed away on April 7, 2017. It has been a difficult one year to processing the death of Mother. I' m just taking one day at a time. In my mind, I'm thinking what we can do to pay tribute to Mother. So, I thought it would be great if all of my siblings would travel back to Greer to pay tribute to Mother, everyone has made plans to travel back to pay tribute to Mother on the following days, April 6- 8th.

We have plan to celebration in her memory. On Friday, April 6th we are planning something special to celebration Mother's memory. Saturday, April 7th the first anniversary of Mother's passing, we will go to the gravesite for a day of remembrance. April 8th, our plans were to attend Mother's home church Bethel UM Church for Sunday service, after which we will all fellowship together for dinner, before someone of us travel back to our homes. We thank God for our Mother Alma Parks Mills the life that she lived and the legacy that she has left behind.

Tribute to Mother's Memory

April 7, 2019, 2nd year

This is the second year of Mother's anniversary, not much has changed. I'm still in a depressed state. Once again I'm preparing to travel back home, for the anniversary of Mother's passing. I'm still not sleeping well. I'm thinking it's going to get back in time. This year the anniversary would only include my two sisters and Dad. We send to the gravesite and send some balloon up and a tribute. It was a low-key event this year. When I visit I'm still having fastback, remembering the day she passed away. It's so difficult looking into the closet when all of her clothes and belongs are. No one wants to clear out her personal belongs. This make the healing process harder, because nothing has changed, it as if Mother is missing but her belongs are still in place.

Tribute of Mother's Memory

April 7, 2020, 3rd year

Not much has changed with the grieving process. It's still a struggle, but I'm trying to stay business so that I won't focus of Mother's death. This year was extremely hard, because of Covid. No one was allowed to travel, due to the pandemic. I did set up a memorial of Mother, with a picture. I still feel sad sometimes. I do try to push those my pain.

Tribute to Mother's Memory

April 7, 2021, 4th year

These years have passed by some quickly. It feels like I'm stuck in a time tunnel. I'm still traveling back to Greer to honor the memory of my Mother anniversary of her death. I do also have a special time to celebrate my Father's birthday. It won't ever be easy to accept her death. But each year is a new beginning. I thought that I would be closer to moving on. Mother is in a better place. I just miss her more and more each year. I do have so many things to be thankful. I do start to feel some stress when it's time for me to plan my annual trip home. Losing someone is along healing process. I do pray to God, that one day I will reach that place.

Tribute to Mother's Memory

April 7, 2022, 5th year

Where did the time go? Time does move on quickly. I have had challenges during these pass five years. Suffering with depression, and feeling the need to talk to Mother. I still don't sleep well, but I know that deep down its time for me to let go. It doesn't seem like Mother has been gone for five years. I can recall it, like it was yesterday. I will travel to Greer, SC, my hometown to visit family. We are planning again for the last five years a gravesite ceremony with my Dad and of my siblings. As I count down to this month marks the five years. I'm still having anxiety leading up to the anniversary this year, I know that things will get better. I know that Mother is smiling down on us, that we have kept her memories going. I don't know what the next chapter will be in my life, but it's time to make a change. I need to focus on the present not the past. Finishing my book has been a healing for me. I can and I will take charge of my life. I thank my daughter Kisha for all of her support. She encouraged me keep moving, and that what I'm going to do.

Chapter 8: Missing Her

Why does the pain of losing a loved one hurt so bad? I miss Mother so much. One thing that was so different was to see Mother change right before my eyes. It first it wasn't too back. But as each stage progressed it became to0 much for me to handle. Each time I came back to she Mother, I just want to cry. It's hard to see you loves suffer. As I got the last stage of her life, it was difficult to see her cry and the depression what so hard for me. I have been close to Mother, that's why it hurts so bad.

No one told me that the pain of losing Mother would be so difficult. It's has been also a year since she left me. I think of her every day. I have lost many loves one, but nothing can compare to how I really feel about this loss. The pain is unbearable; I'm not sleeping well anymore. Somedays, it's really difficult to get my day started. It has been said that in time things will get better. I pray, I read my bible, I attend church, but I still feel empty inside. I dare not question God why this disease came upon my Mother.

As I reflect back in time, I recall traveling back home to see Mother, over the last fifty years since I left home in nineteen hundred and sixty-seven. The worst time was when I returned back to Maryland. Most of the time, I tried not to worry about Mother. I called often to check on her almost every other day. Every time I returned back to Maryland, I would feel sad, and wish I never had to leave her. I tried not to feel guilty when I left my husband. I did what I had to do.

As time went by, Mother's condition was getting worst I would ask my husband when I left the house to run errands, if I received any calls. I would say most days, no news is good news. The grief started for me many years ago when Mother was first diagnosed with dementia. Waiting was the worst part of Mother's illness. Most of the time, I just blocked everything out. I tried to carry on each day as normal as I could.

It has been a great loss for me, losing my Mother, friend, and the love of my life. It feels like a piece of my heart has been taken out of my chest. The grief for my Mother started many years ago, when she was first diagnosed with dementia. It was like watching time on a clock, ticking away. Once the clock stops you knew it would be all over. All I wanted to do was to be by my Mother's side 24/7, but that was impossible since I have a family in Maryland. I decided to travel back to see Mother as much as I could. On some days all I wanted to do was cry, but most of the time I kept it together.

Most of the time I would call home every week, sometimes two to three times. On the day Mother passed away I was there by her bed side. I held up during Mother's home going service. It was if I was in a zone. I blocked everything and everyone out. I didn't see most of my friends and classmates until they walked up to me until the service was over.

At first I was doing great, at least that's what I thought. It's if something triggered my emotions. When my daughters ask me to record the information, I didn't realize how difficult it was going to be. Sometimes, I feel like just screaming to the top of my voice. I'm trying my best to move forward, but it's not working yet. There is a saying that this too shall pass. It's so important to know when to seek help, so I decide to speech with a therapist. During the last weeks or so, it has been difficult for me. Someday I feel so depressed. It's difficult for me to get my day started. My heart feels so heavy. How long will this grief last? I don't want to go anywhere. It's hard for me to concentrate on anything. I pray each day that God will give me the will to keep moving. In time, it will get better.

Losing a loved one to Dementia: How I really feel about the loss of my Mother?

Words can express how I really feel about my loss. No one could have prepared me, for what my life would be like once she was gone. To sum it up, getting educated about the stages of Dementia is very important. Many years ago, I made a promise to visit as much as I could, to be with Mother. We had a close relationship. Before I started my family, I would travel with them. I just felt like, I needed to be around them as much as I could. I really knew that as shed got older, it would be difficult to face the reality of losing her. Sometimes, I feel like it's not fair, but don't know how long we have left on this earth.

Chapter 9: Love Poem for Mother

A Love Poem for Mother

Love is patient, love is kind. It does not envy,

It does not boast it is not proud

1Corinthians 13:4 -NIV

Love is tender, love is sweet.

I'll keep that love until we met.

I know that you are gone and it's so hard.

No one will ever take your place.

Our love was so deep, so I'll always keep you in this

heart.

You were an inspiration, and shared your heart to many.

My heart aches, but no one shall ever take your place.

You were my sweet Mom.

I'll always love you forever.

With all my Love Daughter

Gloria

Chapter 10: A Song Tribute for Mother

Oh God how do I mend my broken heart?

I will lift up mine eyes unto the hills, from whence

cometh my help.

My Help cometh from the Lord, which made heaven

and earth Psalm 121 1-2

I can think of the years when you were still here

You were everything that I want to be

If I could only see you again

But no one told me about all the sadness that I would

feel

And Oh God how can you mend this broken heart?

Oh God how can I stop the tears from falling down my

face?

What makes this grieve go away?

Oh God how can I keep this broken heart, from break-

ing into?

Oh God, how can I get through this death?

I won't see you tomorrow, oh how I miss you so

I must hold on to the memories of years gone by

Oh God, Only you can mend my broken heart

Chapter 11: A Daughter's Prayer to God

February 18, 2022

Dear God,

Thank you for ninety-one years you gave Mother to us. Please help me understand why. I'm praying for peace and understanding. Help me to live each day to the fullest. Tomorrow isn't promise, so I will enjoy life. I know it was time for Mother to go, but I really didn't want her to go. Was I being selfish? It's so hard to let someone go that you have known them all of your life. God help me to take control of my life. Let me continue to be faithful to your word. Help me to understand why Mother came down with this disease. I do pray for a curse one day for Dementia /Alzheimer disease.

Help me not to worry about coming down with the disease too. Do I really want to know if I have the gene? Let me be a light for someone else's family who may be going through what I have gone through with this life ending disease that has taken my Mother from me. Teach me just to take one day at a time.

In the name of Jesus,
Gloria L. Mills Battle

Chapter 12: Letter to Mother

(Alma Parks Mills)

February 22, 2022

Dear Mother,

I know that you didn't mean to break my heart by leaving me, but I miss you so much. I cried many tears leading up to your death. It's now almost the fifth anniversary of your death. In the beginning I had many depressed days and sleepless nights. On the weeks leading up to your death, I recall telling you that I loved you, while you were lying this in a coma. In my heart I knew that you already knew, but it brought so much love to my heart when you answered back.

I often see you in my dreams that make me feel like you're still with me. I really don't understand the dreams, but I'm always happy to see you. I will always love you with all of my heart. You worked some hard to make sure that I had what I needed. I know that you really want me to move on, but I just still can't let you go. I know that one day, but not too soon we will meet again.

If you were here you would tell me to trust God and to live one day at a time, as you often told me when you were here. Mother it's still hard for me to visit your gravesite when I travel back to Greer. But on a good day, I do well most of the time. You brought me so much joy in my life. I miss seeing your face and home cooked meals, especially your macaroni and cheese, your stuffing during Thanksgiving and other holidays. That Sunday dinner was the best.

Mother you would be so happy to know that I still visiting Dad almost every birthday. He still looks great at ninety-nine years young. When you left us we are stilling trying to hold it together. Yes, we still fight, but the best part is that we always remember that you would want us to still love each other. Tell all of my relatives and family member's hello for me. Rest on in Paradise Mother.

Love your daughter,

Gloria Mills Battle

Chapter 13: What is Alzheimer's /Dementia?[i]

Alzheimer's is a type of dementia that causes problems with memory thinking and behavior. Symptoms usually develop slowly and get worse over time, becoming severe enough to interfere with daily tasks. Alzheimer's is the most common form of dementia, a general term for memory loss and other cognitive abilities serious enough to interfere with daily life. Alzheimer's disease accounts for 60 to 80 percent of dementia cases. Alzheimer's is not a normal part of aging. The greatest known risk factor is increasing age, and the majority of people with Alzheimer's are 65 and older.

But Alzheimer's is not just a disease of old age. Approximately 200, 000 Americans under the age of 65 have younger-onset Alzheimer's disease (also known as early-onset Alzheimer's) Alzheimer's worsen over time. Alzheimer's is a progressive disease, where dementia symptoms gradually worsen over a number of years. In these early stages, memory loss is mild, but with late stage of Alzheimer's individuals lose the ability to carry a conversation and respond to their environment. Alzheimer's is the sixth leading cause of death in the United States.

Those with Alzheimer's live an average of eight years after their symptoms become noticeable to others, but survival can range from four to 20 years, depending on age and other health conditions. Alzheimer's have no current cure, but treatments for symptoms are available and research continues. If you or a loved one has been diagnosed with Alzheimer's or a related dementia, you are not alone. The Alzheimer's Association is the trusted resource for reliable information, education, referral, and support to millions of people affected by the disease.

Chapter 14: Seven Stages of Dementia

Dealing with the Seven Stage of Dementia

- One of the most difficult things to hear about dementia is that, in most cases, dementia is irreversible and incurable. However, with an early diagnosis and proper care, the progression of some forms of dementia can be managed and slowed down. The cognitive decline that accompanies dementia conditions does not happen all at once - the progression of dementia can be divided into seven distinct, identifiable stages.

- Learning about the stages of dementia can help with identifying signs and symptoms early on, as well as assisting sufferers and caretakers in knowing what to expect in further stages. The earlier dementia is diagnosed, the sooner treatment can start. Source: Article taken from website: **Dementia.org**

*I wanted to share this information and articles for persons who may be dealing with a family member, friend, or other persons in your community. Mother was diagnosed early. I notice some changes in Mother. I thought it was her just getting older. I wasn't sure. Thank God we did get her to the doctor to be diagnosed. The best thing that you or your family member can do is to educate yourself about the disease that you are dealing with. I has been there it's extremely for my entire family to have dealt with Mother having dementia. Just being there as she went through the seven stages are unbearable.

One must show patience, and get help with for your loved ones when they need it. I have included an article about; what is dementia? I have included the seven stages of dementia. I will do my best to give you an example of how each stage of dementia affected Mother; I hope that this information will help anyone who may be going through dementia with your loved ones. I hope that this book will give you an insight about dealing with grief, depression, and sadness of losing a Mother, and a loved one.

Stage One, Two & Three of Dementia:

Stage 1: No Cognitive Decline

- Stage 1 of dementia can also be classified as the normal functioning stage. At this stage of dementia development, a patient generally does not exhibit any significant problems with memory, or any cognitive impairment. Stages 1-3 of dementia progression are generally known as "pre-dementia" stages.

Stage 2: Age Associated Memory Impairment

- This stage features occasional lapses of memory most frequently seen in:
- Forgetting where one has placed an object
- Forgetting names that were once very familiar
- Oftentimes, this mild decline in memory is merely normal age-related cognitive decline, but it can also be one of the earliest signs of degenerative dementia. At this stage, signs are still virtually undetectable through clinical testing. Concern for early onset of dementia should arise with respect to other symptoms.

Stage 3: Mild Cognitive Impairment

- Clear cognitive problems begin to manifest in stage 3. A few signs of stage 3 dementia include:
- Getting lost easily
- Noticeably poor performance at work
- Forgetting the names of family members and close friends
- Difficulty retaining information read in a book or passage
- Losing or misplacing important objects
- Difficulty concentrating
- Patients often start to experience mild to moderate anxiety as these symptoms increasingly interfere with day-to-day life. Patients who may be in this stage of dementia are encouraged to have a clinical interview with a clinician for proper diagnosis. **Dementia.org**

Stage Four of Dementia

Stage 4: Mild Dementia

- At this stage, individuals may start to become socially withdrawn and show changes in personality and mood.

Denial of symptoms as a defense mechanism is commonly seen in stage 4. Behaviors to look for include:

- Decreased knowledge of current and/or recent events
- Difficulty remembering things about one's personal history
- Decreased ability to handle finances, arrange travel plans, etc.
- Disorientation
- Difficulty recognizing faces and people
- In stage 4 dementia, individuals have no trouble recognizing familiar faces or traveling to familiar locations. However, patients in this stage will often avoid challenging situations in order to hide symptoms or prevent stress or anxiety.

Stage Five of Dementia

Stage 5: Moderate Dementia

- Patients in stage 5 need some assistance in order to carry out their daily lives. The main sign for stage 5 dementia is the inability to remember major details such as the name of a close family member or a home address. Patients may become disoriented about the time and place, have trouble making decisions, and forget basic information about themselves, such as a telephone number or address.

- While moderate dementia can interfere with basic functioning, patients at this stage do not need assistance with basic functions such as using the bathroom or eating. Patients also still have the ability to remember their own names and generally the names of spouses and children.

Stage Six of Dementia

Stage 6: Moderately Severe Dementia

- When the patient begins to forget the names of their children, spouse, or primary caregivers, they are most likely entering stage 6 of dementia and will need full time care. In the sixth stage, patients are generally unaware of their surroundings, cannot recall recent events, and have skewed memories of their personal past. Caregivers and loved ones should watch for:
- Delusional behavior
- Obsessive behavior and symptoms
- Anxiety, aggression, and agitation

- Loss of willpower

- Patients may begin to wander, have difficulty sleeping, and in some cases will experience hallucinations.

Stage Seven of Dementia

Stage 7: Severe Dementia

- Along with the loss of motor skills, patients will progressively lose the ability to speak during the course of stage 7 dementia. In the final stage, the brain seems to lose its connection with the body. Severe dementia frequently entails the loss of all verbal and speech abilities. Loved ones and caregivers will need to help the individual with walking, eating, and using the bathroom.

- By identifying the earliest stages of dementia as they occur, you may be able to seek medical treatment quickly and delay the onset of later stages. Though most cases of dementia are progressive, some may be reversible, and sometimes dementia-like conditions may be caused by treatable underlying deficiencies or illnesses. The more aware you are of these stages, the quicker you will be able to react and seek help, either for yourself or for a loved one. **Source**: Global Deterioration Scale for Assessment of Primary Degenerative Dementia

*The seven stages of the dementia was the end of Mother's Journey. Mother suffered with dementia for nine years, two more years than the doctors predicated. I do pray the information that I have included in my book will help you and your loves one understand the stages of dementia. There are several websites that you can find helpful information. https://www.Alz.org

Chapter 15: Three Stages of Grief

The three (3) stages of grief

Stage 1: Denial

In some way I was in denial. I thought at first, could this be a mistake. When I would go to visit, I would ask Mom questions to see if she could answer them. At first everything seems so normal. It was still hard to believe that Mom had Dementia; I guess that was my state of denial.

Stage 2: Depression

I can relate to depression after a loss one is gone. For years I want suffered with depression. But when my Mother pass a way the depression got worst. I wasn't able to get a full night's sleep. My sleeping issues are due my depression. I have slept will since my Mother passed away five years ago. Some days, I didn't want to leave home. It was difficult to focus on much of anything. In time my depression will get better. It has been almost five years and I'm still struggling with depression. Most days I can snap out of it. Early on I did speak with my doctor to see if I needed med's. Now I'm dealing with my depression the natural way. Each day you have to count it a blessing if you're handling it great on any given day.

Stage 3: Acceptance

This is the area that I really need help. It has been difficult accepting the death of Mother. I just haven't let it go yet. I'm working on that part of the three stages of grief. Most of the time, when I'm preparing to go South, I get depressed. One of my acceptance processes is visiting Mother's gravesite. Just recent I have been to accept it death. Hopefully each year that passes will get better. I do believe that if Mother could tell me anything, she would say, it's time for me to move on and enjoy my life. I think it time; I pray that I will get some closure soon.

- Denial: When you first learn of a loss, it's normal to think, "This isn't happening." You may feel shocked or numb. This is a temporary way to deal with the rush of overwhelming emotion. It's a defense mechanism.
- Anger: As reality sets in, you're faced with the pain of your loss. You may feel frustrated and helpless.

These feelings later turn into anger. You might direct it toward other people, a higher power, or life in general. To be angry with a loved one who died and left you alone is natural, too.

- Bargaining: During this stage, you dwell on what you could've done to prevent the loss. Common thoughts are "If only..." and "What if..." You may also try to strike a deal with a higher power.

- Depression: Sadness sets in as you begin to understand the loss and its effect on your life. Signs of depression include crying, sleep issues, and a decreased appetite. You may feel overwhelmed, regretful, and lonely.

- Acceptance: In this final stage of grief, you accept the reality of your loss. It can't be changed. Although you still feel sad, you're able to start moving forward with your life.

Source: *What are the stages of grief?*

Medical reviewed by: Dr. Carol De Sarkissian

November 9. 2020

Chapter 16: Guide to Grief

Bereavement: Grieving the Loss of a Loved One

Bereavement is the grief and mourning experience following the death of someone important to you. While it's an inevitable part of life—something that virtually all of us go through at some point—losing someone you love can be one of the most painful experiences you'll ever have to endure.

Whether it's a close friend, spouse, partner, parent, child, or other relative, the death of a loved one can feel overwhelming. You may experience waves of intense and very difficult emotions, ranging from profound sadness, emptiness, and despair to shock, numbness, guilt, or regret. You might rage at the circumstances of your loved one's death—your anger focused on yourself, doctors, other loved ones, or God. You may even find it difficult to accept the person is really gone, or struggle to see how you can ever recover and move on from your loss.

Bereavement isn't limited to emotional responses, either. Grief at the death of a loved one can also trigger physical reactions, including weight and appetite changes, difficulty sleeping, aches and pains, and an impaired immune system leading to illness and other health problems. The level of support you have around you, your personality, and your own levels of health and well-being can all play a role in how grief impacts you following bereavement. But no matter how much pain you're in right now, it's important to know that there are healthy ways to cope with the anguish and come to terms with your grief. While life may never be quite the same again, in time you can ease your sorrow, start to look to the future with hope and optimism, and eventually move forward with your life.

Understanding the grief of losing a loved one intensity of your feelings often depends on the circumstances of your loved one's death, how much time you spent anticipating their loss, your relationship to them, and your previous experiences of bereavement. Of course, just as no two relationships are the same, no two losses are ever the same, either.

In short, the more significant the person was in your life and the more feelings you had for them—regardless of their relationship to you—the greater the impact their loss is likely to have.

Losing a parent

Even as an adult child, losing a parent can be extremely distressing. It's easy to feel lost and for all those old childhood insecurities to suddenly return. You may gain some solace if your parent had a long and fulfilling life, but their death can also cause you to consider your own mortality. If you've lost both parents, you're suddenly part of the older generation, a generation without parents, and you're left to grieve your youth as well. And if your relationship with your parent wasn't an easy one, their death can leave you wrestling with a host of conflicting emotions.

Grieving your loss

Whatever your relationship to the person who died, it's important to remember that we all grieve in different ways. There's no single way to react. When you lose someone important in your life, it's okay to feel how you feel. Some people express their pain by crying, others never shed a tear—but that doesn't mean they feel the loss any less.

Don't judge yourself, think that you should be behaving in a different way, or try to impose a timetable on your grief. Grieving someone's death takes time. For some people, that time is measured in weeks or months, for others it's in years.

Allow yourself to feel. The bereavement and mourning process can trigger many intense and unexpected emotions. But the pain of your grief won't go away faster if you ignore it. In fact, trying to do so may only make things worse in the long run. To eventually find a way to come to terms with your loss, you'll need to actively face the pain. As bereavement counselor and writer Earl Grollman put it, "The only cure for grief is to grieve."

Grief doesn't always move through stages. You may have read about the different "stages of grief"—usually denial, anger, bargaining, depression, and acceptance. However, many people find that grief following the death of a loved one isn't nearly that predictable. For some, grief can come in waves or feel more like an emotional rollercoaster. For others, it can move through some stages but not others.

Don't think that you should be feeling a certain way at a certain time.

Coping with Grief and Loss

Prepare for painful reminders. Some days the pain of your bereavement may seem more manageable than others. Then a reminder such as a photo, a piece of music, or a simple memory can trigger a wave of painful emotions again. While you can't plan ahead for such reminders, you can be prepared for an upcoming holiday, anniversary, or birthday that may reignite your grief. Talk to other friends and family ahead of time and agree on the best ways to mark such occasions.

Moving on doesn't mean forgetting your loved one. Finding a way to continue forward with your life doesn't mean your pain will end or your loved one will be forgotten. Most of us carry our losses with us throughout life; they become part of who we are. The pain should gradually become easier to bear, but the memories and the love you had for the person will always remain.

Need to talk to someone?

Get affordable online counseling from BetterHelp or visit HelpGuide's directory for free helplines and crisis resources. HelpGuide is reader supported. We may receive a commission if you sign up for BetterHelp through the provided link. Learn more.

Seek support

When you lose someone you love, it's normal to want to cut yourself off from others and retreat into your shell. But this is no time to be alone. Even when you don't feel able to talk about your loss, simply being around other people who care about you can provide comfort and help ease the burden of bereavement.

Reaching out to those who care about you can also be an important first step on the road to healing. While some friends and relatives may be uncomfortable with your grief, plenty of others will be eager to lend support. Talking about your thoughts and feelings won't make you a burden. Rather, it can help you make sense of your loved one's death and find ways to honor their memory.

Lean on friends and family. Even those closest to you can struggle to know how to help during a time of bereavement, so don't hesitate to tell others what you need— whether it's helping with funeral arrangements or just being around to talk. If you don't feel you have anyone you can lean on for support at this difficult time, look to widen your social network and build new friendships.

Focus on those who are "good listeners". When you're grieving the loss of a close friend or family member, the most important thing is to feel heard by those you confide in. But the raw emotion of your grief can make some people very uncomfortable. That discomfort can cause them to avoid you, say thoughtless or hurtful things, or lose patience when you talk about your loss. Don't use their actions as a reason to isolate, though. Turn to those who are better able to listen and provide comfort.

Join a bereavement support group. Even when you have support from those closest to you, family and friends may not always know the best ways to help. Sharing your grief with others who have experienced similar losses can help you feel less alone in your pain. By listening to others share their stories, you can also gain valuable coping tips. To find a support group in your area, contact nearby hospitals, funeral homes, or counseling centers, or call a bereavement hotline listed below.

Talk to a bereavement counselor. If you're struggling to accept your loss or your grief feels overwhelming, try talking to a bereavement or grief therapist—in-person or via video conferencing online. Confiding in a professional can help you work through emotions that may be too difficult to share with family or friends, deal with any unresolved issues from your loved one's death, and find healthier ways to adapt to life following your loss.

Draw comfort from your religion. If you're religious, the specific mourning rituals of your faith can provide comfort and draw you together with others to share your grief. Attending religious services, reading spiritual texts, praying, meditating, or talking to a clergy member can also offer great comfort and help you derive meaning from your loved one's death.

To gain some protection on Facebook, for example, you can opt to create a closed group rather than a public page. This means people have to be approved by a group member before they can access the memorial. It's also important to remember that while social media can be a useful tool for reaching out to others, it can't replace the face-to-face support you need at this time.

Celebrate your loved one's life

Rituals such as a funeral or memorial service can fulfill important functions, allowing you to acknowledge and reflect on the person's passing, remember their life, and say goodbye. In the period after a funeral, however, your grief can often become even more intense. Often, other people may appear to have moved on, while you're left struggling to make sense of your "new normal".

Remembering your loved one doesn't have to end with the funeral, though. Finding ways of celebrating the person you loved can help maintain their memory and provide comfort as you move through the grieving process.

Keep a journal or write a letter to your loved one. Saying the things, you never got to say to your loved one in life can provide an important emotional release and help you make sense of what you're feeling.

Create a memorial. Building a memorial to your loved one, creating a website or blog, or compiling a photo album or scrapbook to highlight the love you shared can help promote healing. Planting flowers or a tree in your loved one's memory can be particularly rewarding, allowing you to watch something grow and flourish as you tend to it.

Build a legacy. Starting a campaign or fundraiser in your loved one's name, volunteering for a cause that was important to them, or donating to a charity they supported, for example, can help you find meaning in their loss. It can also add a sense of purpose as you move forward with your own life.

Continue to do things you used to do together. Perhaps you used to go to sports events with your loved one, listen to music, or take long walks together? There's comfort in routine, so when it's not too painful, continuing to do these things can be a way to mark your loved one's life.

Remember your loved one in simple ways. Even simple acts such as lighting a candle, visiting a favorite place, or marking an important date can help the healing process.

Take care of yourself

When you're grieving the death of a loved one, it's easy to neglect your own health and welfare. But the stress, trauma, and intense emotions you're dealing with at the moment can impact your immune system, affect your diet, and sleep, and take a heavy toll on your overall mental and physical health.

Neglecting your well-being may even prolong the grieving process and make you more susceptible to depression or complicated grief. You'll also find it harder to provide comfort to children or other vulnerable family members who are also grieving. However, there are simple steps you can take to nurture your health at this time.

Manage stress. It's probably the last thing you feel like doing at the moment, but exercising is a powerful antidote to stress—and can help you sleep better at night. Relaxation techniques such as deep breathing, meditation, and yoga are also effective ways to ease anguish and worry.

Spend time in nature. Immersing yourself in nature and spending time in green spaces can be a calming, soothing experience when you're grieving. Try gardening, hiking, or walking in a park or woodland.

Pursue interests that enrich your life. Hobbies, sports, and other interests that add meaning and purpose to your life can bring a comforting routine back to your life following the upheaval of bereavement. They can also help connect you with others and nurture your spirit.

Eat and sleep well. Eating a healthy diet and getting enough rest at night can have a huge impact on your ability to cope with grief. If you're struggling to sleep at this difficult time, there are supplements and sleep aids that may be able to help—just try not to rely on them for too long.

Avoid using alcohol or drugs to cope. While it's tempting to use substances to help numb your grief and self-medicate your pain, in the long run excessive alcohol and drug use will only hamper your ability to grieve. Try using HelpGuide's free Emotional Intelligence Toolkit as a healthier way to manage your emotions. When the pain of bereavement doesn't ease up.

You may never truly get over the death of someone you love. But as time passes, it's normal for difficult emotions such as sadness or anger to gradually ease as you begin to accept your loss and move forward with your life. However, if you aren't feeling better over time, or your pain is getting worse, it may be a sign that your grief has developed into a more serious problem, such as complicated grief or major depression.

Grief vs. depression

Distinguishing between grief and depression isn't always easy as they share many symptoms, but there are ways to tell the difference:

Grief can be a roller coaster. It involves a wide variety of emotions and a mix of good and bad days. Even when you're in the middle of the grieving process, you will still have moments of pleasure or happiness.

With **depression**, on the other hand, the feelings of emptiness and despair are constant. Other symptoms that suggest depression, not just grief, include:

- Intense, pervasive sense of guilt.
- Thoughts of suicide or a preoccupation with dying.
- Feelings of hopelessness or worthlessness.
- Slow speech and body movements.
- Inability to function at home, work, or school.
- Seeing or hearing things that aren't there.

What is complicated grief?

While the sadness of losing someone you love never goes away completely, it shouldn't remain center stage. If the pain of the loss is so constant and severe that it keeps you from resuming your life, you may be suffering from a condition known as *complicated grief* or *persistent complex bereavement disorder*.

Complicated grief is like being stuck in an intense state of mourning. You may have trouble accepting the death long after it has occurred or be so preoccupied with the person who died that it disrupts your daily routine and undermines your other relationships.

Symptoms of complicated grief include:

- Intense longing and yearning for your deceased loved one.
- Intrusive thoughts or images of the person.
- Denial of the death or sense of disbelief.
- Imagining that your loved one is alive.
- Searching for the deceased in familiar places.

- Avoiding things that remind you of your loved one.

- Extreme anger or bitterness over your loss.

- Feeling that life is empty or meaningless.

Complicated grief and trauma

If your loved one's death was sudden, violent, or otherwise extremely stressful or disturbing, complicated grief can manifest as psychological trauma or PTSD.
Being traumatized from the loss of a loved one can leave you feeling helpless and struggling with upsetting emotions, memories, and anxiety that won't go away. But with the right guidance, you can make healing changes and move on with your life.

Finding professional help

If you're experiencing symptoms of complicated grief, trauma, or clinical depression, talk to a mental health professional right away. Left untreated, these conditions can lead to significant emotional damage, life-threatening health problems, and even suicide. But treatment can help you get better.

Contact a bereavement counselor or therapist if you:

1. Feel like life isn't worth living.
2. Wish you had died with your loved one.
3. Blame yourself for the loss or for failing to prevent it.
4. Feel numb and disconnected for more than a few weeks.
5. Are having difficulty trusting others since your loss.
6. Are unable to perform your normal daily activities.

Authors: Lawrence Robinson and Melinda Smith, M.A.

Last updated: October 2021

References

Get more help

- Grief and Loss – A guide to preparing for and mourning the death of a loved one. (Harvard Medical School Special Health Report)
- Death and Grief – Article for teens on how to cope with grief and loss. (TeensHealth)

- Grief: Coping with Reminders after a Loss – Tips for coping with the grief that can resurface even years after you've lost a loved one. (Mayo Clinic)
- Life after Loss: Dealing with Grief – Guide to coping with grief and loss. (University of Texas Counseling and Mental Health Center)
- Bereavement – Symptoms, causes, and treatment. (Psychology Today)
- Bereavement and Grief – Mourning the loss of a loved one. (Mental Health America)
- Understanding Grief – Articles to help you cope with the grieving process. (Cruse Bereavement Care)

Bereavement resources

Helplines:

In the U.S.: Crisis Call Center at 775-784-8090

Other support:

- Find a GriefShare group meeting near you – Worldwide directory of support groups for people grieving the death of a family member or friend. (GriefShare)

- Find Support – Directory of programs and support groups in the U.S. for children experiencing grief and loss. (National Alliance for Grieving Children)
- Chapter Locator for finding help for grieving the loss of a child in the U.S. and International Support for finding help in other countries. (The Compassionate Friends)

If you're feeling suicidal...

Seek help immediately. Please read Suicide Help, talk to someone you trust, or call a suicide helpline:

- In the U.S., call 1-800-273-8255.
- Or visit IASP to find a helpline in your country.

Notes

References

All references can be found within the text as listed. The author claims no liability in the usage of additional resources nor privately receive any sponsorship compensation for sharing information on grief and loss.

---

[i] Source: Alz.org/ Alzheimer's Association 24/7 Helpline: 800.272.3900

www.ingramcontent.com/pod-product-compliance
Lightning Source LLC
Chambersburg PA
CBHW070300290526
45791CB00003B/1017